SCIENCE & HOMOEOPATHY

Parallels in the Genetics of Criminal and Antisocial Behaviour

FIONA SPENCER THOMAS LCH

STA BOOKS London

First published in 2015 by STA Books, London

www.spencerthomasassociates.com

ISBN-13: 978-1508922377 (CreateSpace-Assigned)

ACKNOWLEDGEMENTS

I should like to thank my wonderful homoeopath and author, Colin Griffith MCH, for encouraging me to study homoeopathy and discover the wonderful effects of this gentle, safe and effective form of treatment. The tutors at the former London College of Homoeopathy were inspiring and, for their knowledge and passion, I am most grateful. I would also like to thank all those friends who encouraged me and allowed me to treat them.

Last but not least, I would like to thank my amazing daughter Alice for believing in me. She has learnt so much herself. Thanks too to my late husband John, her father who was so supportive during my challenging studies undertaken while I worked full-time in publishing.

For Alice and John

CONTENTS

INTRODUCTION

The problem of difficult children and particularly those who are likely to become criminals as young people and adults has interested me for a long time. Many reasons may contribute to their behaviour including upbringing, trauma, vaccination, illness, alcohol, drugs and other possible influences. A great number of questions are open to debate, including whether genetic inheritance plays a significantly large role in the pattern of behaviour that results in criminal activities in an individual.

In February 1995 there was considerable media coverage of a London conference organised by The Ciba Foundation in collaboration with The Wellcome Centre for Medical Science. The subject was The Genetics of Criminal and Antisocial Behaviour and the conference was held to air the latest evidence from the scientific community on the possibility of identifying specific genes that affect behaviour.

Presentations were made by six American experts at the Open Meeting under the chairmanship of Professor Sir Michael Rutter of the Institute of Psychiatry, London. These presentations included a survey of twin studies, evidence from adoption surveys, molecular genetic studies, genetics and animal models for human aggression, interpersonal violence: an evolutionary psychological perspective and the legal implications of genetics and crime research (in the USA). Of these, the papers delivered by two of the scientists caught my attention - Dr Michael J Lyons of the Department of Psychology, Boston University, USA, whose work on Twin Studies presents some interesting evidence for the case of genetic association with criminal activity, and that of Dr Sarnoff A Mednick of the Centre for Longitudinal Research, University of Southern California, Los Angeles.

1

It was the results of their research that led me to want to enquire further and discover whether homoeopathic parallels could be drawn between the scientific studies of inherited traits that might be passed down through families, and provide a homoeopathic perspective on the these findings. My hope is that this study might create a bridge between the two schools and suggest ways in which conventional medicine might look at what can be achieved through homoeopathic treatment. For the homoeopath, I hope that the work would present an up-to-date picture of scientific thinking on these two disorders, offering useful background information, as well as pointers to rubrics that might be common to the various internationally identified symptoms of these behavioural abnormalities.

Always bearing in mind that the basis of homoeopathic philosophy is to treat the patient as an individual, I decided to embark on an exploration of the rubrics associated with the different symptoms involved in Conduct Disorder and Antisocial Personality Disorder. My objective was to try and identify a thread of remedies and possible miasms that could assist in the treatment of difficult children likely to become criminals. These disorders are defined in The Diagnostic and Statistical Manual of Mental Disorders (DSMIV).

DSMIV is published by the American Institute of Psychiatry and is an internationally acknowledged publication describing the criteria for the two identified disorders, which are also laid out in the International Classification of Disease (ICD 10), produced by the World Health Organisation, Geneva. The description of Conduct Disorder in the ICD appears under classification F91 - Conduct disorders, and the Antisocial Personality Disorder as F60.2 Dissocial Personality Disorder. According to a spokesman from the Institute of Psychiatry in London, the DSMIV criteria for the two disorders are more widely used, as the symptoms as defined in that publication are more specific.

1

THE EVIDENCE OF SCIENTIFIC RESEARCH AND A PRESENTATION OF HOMOEOPATHIC PHILOSOPHY

Are Behavioural Traits Inherited?

Two conditions appear in the Diagnostic and Statistical Manual of Mental Disorders, fourth edition, which identify a range of criteria from disobedience to borderline or actual criminal behaviour. These are **Conduct Disorder**, usually identified in children up to the age of 15, and **Antisocial Personality Disorder** which is characterised by its appearance after the age of 18. These two disorders are often interrelated and the ages involved in the classification differ according to the specific criteria that are present at any one particular age. The latter also involves a history of Conduct Disorder diagnosed in an individual prior to 15 years of age. For example, an individual over the age of 18 can only be diagnosed as suffering from Conduct Disorder if the criteria for Antisocial Personality Disorder are not also met. However, in both instances the common thread is a persistent pattern of negative behaviour over a long period by the person involved, combined with a lack of feeling or a disregard for the wishes, feelings and rights of others. Another common feature is that both these disorders are markedly prevalent in the male, probably because of the aggressive nature of the identifying symptoms.

There are two sub-types of Conduct Disorder that are based on the age of onset. Childhood onset type is identified when there is a history of at least one symptom prior to the age of 10. This tends to grow to a full Conduct Disorder prior to puberty and evolve into adult Antisocial Personality Disorder.

The criteria laid down for these disorders are set out as described in DSMIV[1] and provide the basis for this study into genetic traits that might lead to criminal behaviour.

---

[1] Reprinted with permission from the Diagnostic and Statistical Manual of Mental Disorders, Fourth Edition, (Copyright ©1994). American Psychiatric Association. All Rights Reserved.

DIAGNOSTIC CRITERIA FOR 312.8
CONDUCT DISORDER

A.

A repetitive and persistent pattern of behaviour in which the basic rights of others or major age-appropriate societal norms or rules are violated, as manifested by the presence of three (or more) of the following criteria in the past 12 months.

AGGRESSION TO PEOPLE AND ANIMALS
1   often bullies, threatens, or intimidates others
2   often initiates physical fights
3   has used a weapon that can cause serious physical harm to others (e.g. a bat, brick, broken bottle, knife, gun)
4   has been physically cruel to people
5   has been physically cruel to animals
6   has stolen while confronting a victim (e.g. mugging, purse snatching, extortion, armed robbery)
7   has forced someone into sexual activity.

DESTRUCTION OF PROPERTY
8   has deliberately engaged in fire setting with the intention of causing serious damage
9   has deliberately destroyed others' property (other than by fire setting)

DECEITFULNESS OR THEFT
10 has broken into someone else's house, building or car
11 often lies to obtain goods or favours or to avoid obligations (i.e. 'cons' others)
12 has stolen items of non-trivial value without confronting a victim (e.g. shoplifting, but without breaking and entering; forgery)

SERIOUS VIOLATIONS OF RULES

13 often stays out at night despite parental prohibitions, beginning before age 13 years
14 has run away from home overnight at least twice while living in parental or parental surrogate home (or once without returning for a lengthy period)
15 is often truant from school, beginning before age 13 years

B.

The disturbance in behaviour causes clinically significant impairment in social, academic or occupational functioning.

C.

If the individual is age 18 years or older, criteria are not met for Antisocial Personality Disorder.

Specify type based on age at onset.

Childhood-Onset Type: onset of at least one criterion characteristic of Conduct Disorder prior to age 10 years

Adolescent-Onset Type: absence of any criteria characteristic of Conduct Disorder prior to age 10 years.

Specify severity:

Mild: few if any conduct problems in excess of those required to make the diagnosis and conduct problems cause only minor harm to others.

Moderate: number of conduct problems and effect on others intermediate between 'mild' and 'severe'

Severe: many conduct problems in excess of those required to make the diagnosis **or** conduct problems cause considerable harm to others.

DIAGNOSTIC CRITERIA FOR 301.7
ANTISOCIAL PERSONALITY DISORDER

A.

There is a pervasive pattern of disregard for and violation of the rights of others occurring since age 15 years, as indicated by three (or more) of the following:

1   failure to conform to social norms with respect to lawful behaviour as indicated by repeatedly performing acts that are grounds for arrest
2   deceitfulness, as indicated by repeated lying, use of aliases, or conning others for personal profit or pleasure
3   impulsiveness or failure to plan ahead
4   irritability and aggressiveness as indicated by repeated physical fights or assaults
5   reckless disregard for safety of self or others
6   consistent irresponsibility, as indicated by repeated failure to sustain consistent work behaviour or honour financial obligations
7   lack of remorse, as indicated by being indifferent to or rationalising having hurt, mistreated or stolen from another

B.

The individual is at least age 18 years.

C.

There is evidence of Conduct Disorder with onset before age 15 years

D.

The occurrence of Antisocial Behaviour is not exclusively during the course of Schizophrenia or a Manic Episode

Looking at the criteria listed here, it is possible to see that many of them may occur as a consequence of contact with another person who suffers from either of these disorders. For example, a child running away from home might do so because of maltreatment such as physical or sexual abuse. Consequently they might become subject to an aroused level of adrenalin, causing a fight or flight state which may result in aggression as a means of providing them with a protective survival strategy. A familial pattern is identified in Antisocial Personality Disorder criteria which states that this disorder is 'more common among the first-degree biological relatives of those with the disorder than among the general population. The risk to biological relatives of females with the disorder tends to be higher than the risk to biological relatives of the males with the disorder'. This does not mirror the statistical evidence which shows a 3% in males and 1% female community spread but, bearing in mind that the woman is usually more involved in the upbringing of a child, this might well provide the added environmental factor to the already present biological trait to warrant this statement.

It is not therefore surprising to learn that statistics gathered from twin and adoption studies suggest that the risk of children with a biological parent suffering from Antisocial Personality Disorder being diagnosed as suffering from Conduct Disorder is increased. The environmental influence is also emphasised in the same study and indicates that adoptive parents with this disorder are also likely to influence a child, as is a sibling.

A paper given by Dr S A Mednick of the Centre for Longitudinal Research at the University of Southern California offered significant evidence drawn from a study in Denmark of 14,427 non-familial adoptions of new born babies during the period 1924-47 by a group of Danish and US scientists studying schizophrenia. They selected those individuals with a record of three or more convictions for criminal offences as the basis for their research. Because the records of adoptees used in the survey were so complete, due to the fact that all those where the biological father could not be positively identified were discarded, the statistics offer what appears to be strong evidence of an hereditary element in criminal behaviour.

The study also looked at the records, where available, of 65,560 members of wider adoption families, i.e. the adoptive parents and the biological parents. Among these, almost 30% of these biological parents had been convicted of a criminal offence and among the biological fathers, there were 10.2% who had two or more convictions.

Taking the newborn infant away from its biological parents removed it from any environmental influences that it may otherwise have gained from that family that might compound the genetic influences. Consequently, it was left with only the possibility of environmentally acquired behaviour from adoptive parents from which to develop any criminal trends.

The results of the survey of these children, deprived of example from their biological parents, showed that sons who contributed most to the conviction records were influenced as indicated below:

		Biological parents convicted?	
		Yes	**No**
Adoptive parents convicted?	**Yes**	24.5%	14.7%
	No	20%	13.5%

These statistics appear to suggest that there is a strong inherent tendency to criminal behaviour and that the convictions of biological parents have a direct correlation with the conviction rates of their sons. However the wider survey came to the conclusion from their extended records that there was a genetic effect influencing property crimes but not on violent crime.

Another interesting statistic relating to women was obtained from a study that looked at the records of 52 mothers who gave birth in jail and 52 control mothers (not in prison). Of the imprisoned group of mothers, 13 of their progeny were later convicted of a crime as opposed to only 1 child in the control group. (Crowe: Genetics and Crime)

Dr Michael J Lyons of the Department of Psychology at Boston University outlined the conclusions that could be drawn from the results of twin studies. He specifically cited those subjects drawn from the Vietnam Era Twin Registry, which included approximately 3200 male twin pairs of which both twins had served in the US military between 1965 and 1975. These observations suggested that adult antisocial behaviour was more influenced by genetic factors than juvenile behaviour. It also indicated that non-violent antisocial behaviour was more hereditary than violent behaviour but that, when violent behaviour was displayed by an adult, this was more likely to be an inherited trait than it would be in a child.

The classification of disease is achieved by identifying a set of symptoms, either behavioural or physical (or both), which results in a diagnosis. Conduct and Antisocial Personality Disorders are diagnosable disorders (or diseases), as is Schizophrenia which mental symptoms sometimes overlap these disorders. (However, there are five identifiable biotypes that constitute the majority of schizophrenics.) Therefore it would be appropriate to cite the research of Franz Kallman whose study of a thousand pairs of affected monozygotic or identical twins demonstrated that there was an 86.2% chance that, if one of the pair was affected by schizophrenia, the other would be also. His findings also showed that there was a 68.1% chance of two affected parents producing a schizophrenic child.

Professor Sir Michael Rutter, Professor of Child and Adolescent Psychiatry at the Institute of Psychiatry, London, denies there is any such thing as a gene for crime. Some years ago there was a suggestion that a chromosome abnormality (XYY) was associated with aggressive behaviour. Although investigations have shown there to be some link, it is not significant. Rather, he insists that behaviour is a response to stress and offers by way of argument, the risk-taking element of many of the identified criteria which could equally be used to positive effect. He also stressed the national differences in crime comparing the UK and US where the murder rate is over twelve times higher among young people, pointing out that this is unlikely to be a genetic factor.

I would suggest that these statistics might indicate a strong acquired factor such as the mass vaccination programme (this will be discussed later) in that country, or even the culture of gun violence on which its youth is reared. One might ponder an idea that may prove controversial, that a country spawned on adventurers, risk takers and escapees from diverse societies and assorted scenarios, not to mention the slaves wrenched from their own cultures, might have created an altogether different kind of person with a higher level of adrenaline than people living in countries that have evolved in situ over many generations. This genetic tendency may have been the result of an acquired miasm (this will be discussed in the pages that follow) by the emigrés which has been passed down to create the more aggressive generation that exists in that country, with its consequent influence on the crime statistics.

This adrenalin-related antisocial behaviour pattern is borne out in an article by Colin Griffith (The Homoeopath, 56, 1995) in which he suggests that 'babies in utero can become hooked on their mothers' adrenaline which might flow in excess because of trauma, fearfulness or over-work'. He goes on to say that 'The excess adrenaline flow, Moro, is frequently found to be still active in maturity' and may manifest as aggression, learning difficulties and abnormal reflexes such as a light response of either an alternately contracting and dilating pupil, or one that cannot contract fully. These are normally seen as reflex responses to fear. This reflex alone can manifest in a brightly lit classroom where it can result in reading and learning difficulties because of the eye's consequent inability to absorb the information correctly. This might contribute to the one-third of antisocial boys who have specific reading difficulties.

The scientific evidence apart, logic would seem to indicate that, as there are accepted genetic aspects to the offspring of any couple, from inherited features to talents and failings with non-physical qualities such as creativity that are able to be enhanced or extinguished by environmental factors, so why not the criminal tendency? It is certainly a dangerous topic to explore, as the results, even though the indications are that there is little evidence for the hereditary element of violent behaviour in children, might conclude that the child of criminal parents could constitute a threat to society, and where does that take the debate?

From a homoeopathic viewpoint there are very strong indications of inherited traits passed down through families. Unlike the scientific evidence which presents the statistical data on parent and child, homoeopathy looks back to the root causes of disease states, whether mental or physical, and their evolution and transmission through family lines. Homoeopathic philosophy embraces the concept of the acquired and environmental factors and through the writings of its founder, Dr Samuel Hahnemann, has arrived at its parallel conclusion which he called the Miasm. In THE ORGANON 78, he refers to 'illness, which through infection or heredity, has profoundly marked them' (the patients) pointing out that these old illnesses can be aroused through negative passions and particularly 'inappropriate medical treatment'. Historically this would relate to the strongly suppressive skin treatments, such as mercury and sulphur, of Hahnemann's age and those against which he railed when he began to move away from his medical training towards his homoeopathic philosophy and practice.

The scientific argument for acquired genes not passed on via the normal sperm/egg route is presented in Richard Dawkins' The Selfish Gene[2] - by permission of Oxford University Press. Using, by way of example, the rabid dog whose personality is changed through the acquisition of the rabies virus and roams far and wide, possessed by this virus and its need to propagate in another host via the saliva, he suggests that this is an alternative route for genes to pass from body to body. Dawkins says 'Both classes' (of genes, inherited or those passing via unorthodox routes i.e. invading parasitic genes) 'may include genes that originated as 'own' chromosomal genes. And both classes may include genes that originated as external, invading parasites.' Interestingly, this reflects the homoeopathic concept of the acquired miasm which is said to be the result of an external influence (e.g. rabies) that changes the state of the host and consequently becomes a part of that host's chromosomal genes, available for transmission to their progeny.

---

[2] The Selfish Gene by Richard Dawkins (1989) reprinted by permission of Oxford University Press

To provide the background for an exploration of the parallels between the scientific and homoeopathic viewpoints, it is necessary to look further into the concept of the miasm.

After years in the successful practice of his homoeopathic method of healing, Hahnemann began to investigate the underlying reasons as to why his well-selected and effective remedies did not always maintain their cure permanently. Some patients seemed to be getting well in the defined and proven ways and then relapsed. This led him to study the underlying reasons as to why the cure had not been completely effective and, at this point, Hahnemann began to ponder the possibility that there must be some deeper disease providing a soil on which the presenting illness could feed.

After a lifelong study into the foundations of disease he identified three basic diseases from which all others appeared to spring. It was, he believed, the suppression of the symptoms of these historic diseases that had caused them to be driven deep into the economy of the patient causing them to manifest as more sinister symptoms, not just in the immediate sufferer's body, but also through their progeny.

These symptoms he identified as the very basic, first chronicled disease of mankind; the itch or scabious eruption, which Hahnemann called PSORA. The second and third of these were the sexually transmitted diseases that were rife throughout the ages, Syphilis and Gonorrhoea. The first he called SYPHILIS and the second SYCOSIS. These might, in fact, have been described as the children of Psora as Hahnemann concluded that they arose from the Psoric Miasm. On these he based his miasmatic theory to which have been added other miasms including Tuberculosis, Cancer and, more recently, Aids. However, it is still possible to return to the three roots of illness and suggest that the others are genetic mutations and amalgamations of the ancient first three.

Apart from the obvious symptoms of the first three miasms identifiable with the original diseases, many other symptoms became apparent in other spheres and, to this end, Hahnemann chronicled the various paths that each miasm could take. Psora tended generally to present as underfunction in all its spheres, Syphilis as a destructive miasm and Sycosis as an over function. The symptoms of these three miasms present in their characteristic ways in the mental state of the individual. A Psoric person would suffer from a low physical energy, although their mental capacity might be high. In the Organon 80, he explains that Psora is 'the only real fundamental cause and producer of all the other numerous forms of disease...' and includes nervous debility, hysteria, mania, madness, imbecility and melancholia. A Syphilitic character would have a tendency to destruction, which in the extreme, could lead to alcohol and substance abuse, cruelty and the kind of depression that might lead to suicide. On the other hand, Sycosis would be indicated in a person who was greedy, overactive and manipulative.

All three miasms can be recognised in the different rubrics that can be associated with the criteria in CONDUCT DISORDER and ANTISOCIAL PERSONALITY DISORDER. The following chart gives an extensive selection of these. Among these rubrics, all the miasms are implicated. In the case of a robbery, to quote Yair Shemmer (homoeopath, Israel), the miasmatic robber might work in this way. The Psoric plans the robbery, the Syphilitic attacks the guards and the Sycotic grabs the cash.

The numbers 1-15 on the column headings relate to the relevant CONDUCT DISORDER SYMPTOMS and those marked with an A next to column headings 1-7 are related to their associated ANTISOCIAL PERSONALITY DISORDERS criteria as listed on pages 12 to 14. The rubrics appear in KENT'S REPERTORY.

15

KENT'S RUBRICS RELATING TO DISORDERS

Rubrics with page numbers	1	A	2	A	3	A	4	A	5	A	6	A	7	A	8	A	9	10	11	12	13	14	15	Total Conduct Dis.	Total Antisocial Pers.Dis.	Total
Abusive - insulting 4	*	*	*		*																			2	1	3
Abusive without being angry 4	*	*	*		*				*															3	2	5
Anger violent 3						*		*	*															3	1	4
Answers - aversion to 3																	*							1		1
Answers incorrectly 3				*													*							1	1	2
Aversion to members of family 9	*	*	*						*		*									*	*			2		2
Audacity 9	*								*		*			*						*	*			2	3	5
Avarice 9			*		*						*								*	*				3	1	4
Battles, talks about 9		*		*			*		*															2	1	3
Biting 9		*					*	*	*							*								3	1	4
Break things, desires to 10					*									*	*	*								3		3
Business, averse to 10						*					*		*									*		1	2	3
Capriciousness 10						*					*									*	*	*		3	2	5
Censorious 10	*					*																		1		1
Chaotic 10													*												2	2
Concentration difficult 13											*		*												1	1
Contemptuous 16	*	*			*				*		*			*	*		*		*	*	*	*	*	8	5	13
Contradict - disposition to 16			*				*		*													*		1	1	2
Contrary 16			*				*				*						*			*	*	*	*	4		4
Courageous 17			*				*				*			*		*			*		*	*	*	5	2	7
Cowardice 17													*												1	1
Cruelty 17							*	*	*	*			*	*					*		*	*		3	2	5
Cut, desires to, others 17				*		*	*	*	*															2	1	3
Deceitful 17		*			*						*		*		*		*		*	*	*	*	*	7	1	8
Defiant 17	*	*	*						*		*		*		*		*		*	*	*	*	*	9	4	13
	1	A	2	A	3	A	4	A	5	A	6	A	7	A	8	A	9	10	11	12	13	14	15	Total Conduct Dis.	Total Antisocial Pers.Dis.	Total

KENT'S RUBRICS RELATING TO DISORDERS

	1	A	2	A	3	A	4	A	5	A	6	A	7	A	8	9	10	11	12	13	14	15	Total Conduct Dis.	Total Antisocial Pers.Dis.	Total
Destructiveness 36	*														*	*	*						3		3
Dictatorial 36		*													*								2		2
Discontented 36				*	*															*	*	*	4	2	6
Discontented with everything 36	*			*	*															*	*	*	4	3	7
Disobedient 37	*		*																	*	*	*	3	2	5
Escape, attempts to 39																				*	*	*	3		3
Escape from family 39																				*	*	*	3		3
Escape, to run away 39																				*	*	*	3		3
Estranged from family 39											*									*	*		2		2
Exertion, aggravation from mental 41					*		*																	2	2
Fights wants to 48		*		*		*		*															2	2	4
Fire, wants to set things on 48	*														*								1		1
Gestures, makes violent 50		*		*		*		*	*		*		*										5	1	6
Godless 50							*		*				*	*	*								3	1	4
Heedless 51		*			*		*		*		*		*		*	*	*	*	*	*	*	*	9	3	12
Impetuous 54					*		*		*		*				*	*	*	*	*	*			6	2	8
Inconstancy 54					*		*						*						*					2	2
Indiscretion 55																		*	*				2		2
Indifference 55	*	*		*		*		*	*	*	*	*	*	*	*	*	*	*	*	*	*	*	13	7	20
Indifference to conscience 55	*	*		*		*		*	*	*	*	*	*	*	*	*	*	*		*	*		11	4	15
Indifference to loved ones 55																				*	*		2		2
Indifference to relations 55																				*	*		2		2
Indifference to suffering 55				*		*		*	*	*	*		*		*	*							7	2	9
Indifference to welfare of others 55	*						*		*		*		*		*	*	*	*	*				11	3	14
Indolence 56																					*	*	1	2	3
Insolent 57	*	*		*					*		*		*	*	*	*		*	*	*	*	*	7	2	9
	1	A	2	A	3	A	4	A	5	A	6	A	7	A	8	9	10	11	12	13	14	15	Total Conduct Dis.	Total Antisocial Pers.Dis.	Total

17

KENT'S RUBRICS RELATING TO DISORDERS

	1	A	2	A	3	A	4	A	5	A	6	A	7	A	8	A	9	10	11	12	13	14	15	Total Conduct Dis.	Total Antisocial Pers.Dis.	Total
Irresolution 57													*				*								2	2
Irritability 57		*	*																						1	1
Kicks 60		*	*						*															2	1	3
Kill, desires to 60				*	*		*		*															1	1	2
Kill, desires to at sight of a knife 60					*		*		*															1	1	2
Kill, sudden impulse to 60		*			*		*		*															2	1	3
Kill, threatens to 61	*				*		*		*															2	1	3
Kleptomania 61	*		*								*	*												3	2	5
Lascivious 61													*											1		1
Lewdness 62													*											1		1
Libertinism 62											*		*											1		1
Lie 62	*	*	*						*															1	2	3
Malicious 63	*	*	*	*	*		*	*	*	*	*	*	*				*	*	*	*				12	5	17
Misanthropy 66	*	*	*	*	*		*	*	*	*	*		*				*	*						5	5	10
Mischievous 63	*	*	*	*	*	*	*	*	*	*	*	*	*				*	*	*	*				11	4	15
Mood changeable 67							*		*								*	*	*						3	3
Moral feeling, want of 68	*	*	*	*	*		*	*	*	*	*	*	*				*	*	*	*				12	4	16
Obstinate 69	*	*	*		*		*		*		*		*							*	*	*		4	3	7
Persists in nothing 69						*							*									*	*	1	2	3
Pull hair, desires to 70			*		*		*		*								*							2	1	3
Quarrelsome 70	*	*	*		*		*		*								*							3	1	4
Quarrelsome without anger 70	*	*	*				*		*								*							3	1	4
Rage when aroused 71													*				*								1	1
Rage violent 71									*		*										*			3	1	4
Rashness 71	*	*	*		*		*		*		*		*				*	*						8	2	10
Reproaches others 71	*	*														*					*			2	1	3
	1	A	2	A	3	A	4	A	5	A	6	A	7	A	8	A	9	10	11	12	13	14	15	Total Conduct Dis.	Total Antisocial Pers.Dis.	Total

KENT'S RUBRICS RELATING TO DISORDERS

	1	A	2	A	3	A	4	A	5	A	6	A	7	A	8	A	9	10	11	12	13	14	15	Total Conduct Dis.	Total Antisocial Pers.Dis.	Total
Repulsive mood 71	*	*	*		*		*		*		*		*		*		*	*	*					11	1	12
Restlessness 72	*	*	*	*	*																			3	2	5
Restlessness in children 73	*		*		*																			3		3
Rudeness 75	*	*																						1	1	2
Runs about 75	*		*		*																			3		3
Sensitiveness, want of 79	*	*	*	*	*	*	*	*	*	*	*		*		*		*	*	*					11	5	16
Shameless 79	*		*																					2		2
Slander, disposition to 81	*	*	*	*	*																			3	2	5
Spits in face of people 82	*	*	*		*																			3	1	4
Striking 84	*	*	*		*		*		*		*													6	1	7
Striking in children 84	*		*		*		*		*															5		5
Tears things 87	*		*																					2		2
Threatening 85	*	*	*	*	*		*		*		*													6	2	8
Throws things at persons 88	*	*	*																					2	1	3
Time, fritters away 88	*	*		*																				1	2	3
Travel, desire to 89	*		*																					2		2
Undertake, lacks will to 91	*	*		*																				1	2	3
Unfeeling 91	*	*	*	*	*	*	*		*		*		*		*		*	*						10	3	13
Untruthful 91	*	*	*	*	*		*																	4	2	6
Violent 91	*	*	*		*		*		*		*		*											7	1	8
Violent deeds, rage leading to 91	*	*	*		*		*		*															5	1	6
Wander, desires to 92	*		*		*																			3		3
Wicked disposition 95	*	*	*	*	*	*	*	*	*		*		*		*		*	*						10	4	14
Wild feeling in head 95	*	*	*	*	*	*	*	*	*															5	4	9
Wildness 95	*	*	*	*	*		*		*															5	2	7
Work aversion to mental 95		*		*																					2	2
Work impossible 95		*		*																					2	2
	1	A	2	A	3	A	4	A	5	A	6	A	7	A	8	A	9	10	11	12	13	14	15	Total Conduct Dis.	Total Antisocial Pers.Dis.	Total

There are other rubrics that might be included such as Hatred 51, or the various deliria and delusions listed below, but it was felt that these were not common enough to the listed criteria to include them in the chart. They would, however, be useful rubrics in individual cases where the symptoms were present.

Delirium
on being aroused 18
erotic 18
exaltation of strength 18
fierce 19
frightful 19
violent 20
wild 20

Delusion
not appreciated 21
he is a criminal 23
there is danger to his life 23
there is danger from family 23
is despised 23
does not belong to family 25
is persecuted 30
is poor 31
separated from the world 31
is repudiated by relatives 31
has suffered wrong 35

The symptoms above would be more likely to appear in the course of a Schizophrenic or Manic episode and these are excluded from the criteria of Antisocial Personality Disorder if they only occur during these episodes.

Clearly there are a few strong characteristics that run through all the given symptoms in the chart. These include:

Contempt
Defiance
Heedlessness
Indifference generally, and specifically, **to conscience, suffering** and **the welfare of others**.
Maliciousness
Mischievousness
Rashness
Repulsive Mood
Want of Sensitiveness
Unfeeling
and
Wicked Disposition

These characteristics describe a person who appears to be isolated and to have a complete lack of awareness or interest in his interaction with society as well as a lack of internal control. Looking at the symptoms here, once again one can see different miasms appearing. To obtain a list of remedies which relate to this hard core of symptoms, the following chart was prepared from the computerised MACREPERTORY. In section 3 the relationship of these remedies to the miasms is explored.

Rubrics	Anac.	Lyc.	Nux-v.	Hyos.	Lach.	Merc.	Phos.	Stram.	Op.	Plat.	Ars.	Nat-m.	Puls.	Bell.	Calc.	Con.	Cupr.	Nit-ac.
Total	15	13	11	10	10	10	10	10	9	9	9	9	9	8	8	8	8	8
Total	7	7	6	6	6	6	6	5	4	5	5	5	5	6	4	6	6	6
1. Mind; CONTEMPTUOUS		2	2	1	1					3	2	1	1					1
2. Mind; DEFIANT	1	2	1									2		1		2		
3. Mind; HEEDLESS	2	2		1	2	2	2		2	1	2	3		2	2	2	1	1
4. Mind; INDIFFERENCE	2	2	1	2	2	2	3	1	3	3			3				1	2
5. Mind; INDIFFERENCE; conscience, to the dictates of								3	3									
6. Mind; INDIFFERENCE; suffering, to																		
7. Mind; INDIFFERENCE; welfare of others, to								3	1									
8. Mind; MALICIOUS	2	2	3	2	2	1	1			1	2	2	2	2	2	1	2	2
9. Mind; MISANTHROPY	2	2		2	1	1	2	2		1		1		1	2	1	1	1
10. Mind; MISCHIEVOUS	3		3	2	2	2					2				2		2	
11. Mind; RASHNESS													1					
12. Mind; REPULSIVE mood		1	1			2	1	1			1		2			1		
13. Mind; SENSITIVE; want of sensitiveness							1							1		1	1	1
14. Mind; UNFEELING	3													1				
15. Mind; WICKED disposition																		

This page is a homeopathic repertory grid. Remedy abbreviations (with their two total figures) head the columns; rubrics are listed as rows.

Rubric	Am-m. 5/4	Verat. 6/4	Ign. 6/5	Hep. 6/4	Gual. 6/6	Caust. 6/5	Bar-c. 6/5	Ambr. 6/5	Agar. 6/4	Ph-ac. 6/3	Nat-c. 7/4	Hell. 7/3	Cic. 7/5	Chin. 7/4	Aur. 7/4	Arn. 7/5	Acon. 7/5	Sulph. 8/5
1. Mind; CONTEMPTUOUS			1		1								3	2				
2. Mind; DEFIANT					1	1										2	1	
3. Mind; HEEDLESS					1	2						2						
4. Mind; INDIFFERENCE	1	1	1	1	1	1	1	1	1	1	1	3	1			2	2	2
5. Mind; INDIFFERENCE; conscience, to the dictates of	1	2	2	1			2	1	2	3	3		1	3				
6. Mind; INDIFFERENCE; suffering, to												2						
7. Mind; INDIFFERENCE; welfare of others, to																		3
8. Mind; MALICIOUS																		1
9. Mind; MISANTHROPY				2	1	1	1	1	1		1		1	1	2	1	2	1
10. Mind; MISCHIEVOUS	1	1	1		1		1	2			2		1		2	1	1	
11. Mind; RASHNESS	2						1		2							1		
12. Mind; REPULSIVE mood														1	2			
13. Mind; SENSITIVE; want of sensitiveness		2		2		1		1		2					1	1	1	1
14. Mind; UNFEELING			1			1		1										
15. Mind; WICKED disposition																		

23

2

ENVIRONMENTAL INFLUENCES ON THE DELINQUENT

"Whatever our genes, we are responsible for our behaviour." Emma Nicholson, Conservative MP on Question Time, BBC 1 (May 1995)

To a certain extent this statement must be correct, but what of those people who have inherited tendencies to criminal behaviour, the feasibility of which has been described in the previous section, or environmentally or acquired behaviours? The latter is a homoeopathically accepted fact, (i.e. as a result of trauma, stress, illness or vaccination).

Homoeopathy acknowledges that a person's health should be viewed as a whole and not as disparate parts. It therefore accepts that abnormal behaviour is related to other changes that may be occurring in the human economy. Homoeopathy also acknowledges that this constitution may be inherited or acquired in a person's lifetime therefore accepting the likelihood of environmental influences affecting the individual. It also suggests that the individual's latent (or active) miasm(s) inherited from their parents, may affect their individual response to stress or disease. Take, for example an epidemic of cholera. Not everyone who comes into contact with the disease will have a susceptibility and those who don't will not contract it. This situation is mirrored in an individual's response to emotional and psychological events.

Looking back at the statistics shown on page 16 which demonstrate that there was almost a 10% increased crime rate in the adopted sons of biological and adoptive parents both convicted of crimes, to those where only the adoptive parents had criminal records. This suggests strongly that the biological urge is playing a very strong part. The difference between the statistics where the biological sons of parents with records had been exposed to criminal influences in their adoptive family was 4.5%, demonstrating that the environmental factor does have an effect in arousing the biological tendency. In the sons of unconvicted biological parents this environmental influence is just over 1%. Clearly, from these figures, the biological influence plays the largest part but the environment is also influential.

The results of a report compiled by Academia Europaea, whose purpose was to review scientific evidence and discover whether psychosocial disorders, including crime, had increased among the young over the past 50 years were announced on May 30th 1995. Coordinated by Professor Sir Michael Rutter and Professor David Smith, Professor of Criminology at Edinburgh University, it offers the conclusion to a five-year study by academics in Europe and the United States.

The findings concluded that recorded crime (most committed by young people) has increased tenfold from 1950 to 1993. Other observations were that there is strong evidence that family conflict and bad parenting increased the risk that children would later develop disorders, but it is uncertain as to whether the rise in divorce is responsible for this. Indications are that the poor, unemployed and people living on run down estates are more likely to be criminal, depressed, suicidal and addicted to drugs than those living in more comfortable surroundings. It also suggests that the mass media is unlikely to be the root cause of the increase of psychosocial disorder although it may have added to negative influences. The report also acknowledges that unfulfilled rising expectations may be among the causes of increasing disorder (Daily Telegraph, May 30, 1995).

To refer once again to a work of Michael Rutter, in his book Helping Troubled Children[3] - ©Penguin Education (UK), Springer (US) - he writes that 'Typically, children with persistent disorders come from families where there is discord and quarrelling; where affection is lacking; where discipline is inconsistent, ineffective and either extremely severe or lax; where the family has broken up through divorce or separation; or where the children have had periods of being placed 'in care' at times of family crisis.' This appears to bear out the report's findings to a certain extent. However, there may be other external influences playing a larger part on the child's psyche in 1995 than was the case in 1975. Today children reach puberty earlier and many experiment with alcohol and substances and consequently their relationship with their families may not be quite as close as was the case two decades ago. Another factor may be that the educational system is extending and children remain financially dependent on their parents for longer. In fact they are in limbo - neither a child, nor an adult. Also they are becoming isolated from the rest of society with their own music, dress and culture.

If, as the report suggests, bad parenting plays a significant role in conduct and antisocial personality disorders, then it reflects the conclusions of the DSM criteria and indicates a stronger likelihood of perpetuity through generations, as a consequence of a learned behaviour pattern, as well as inherited behaviour.

This same report draws attention to what a homoeopath would read as understood. 'This is the first major study to highlight the upward trend in psychosocial disorders of youth

---

[3] HELPING TROUBLED CHILDREN by Michael Rutter (Penguin Books 1990)
Copyright © Michael Rutter, 1976, 1990

since the Second World War. It is striking that this increase happened at a time when physical health was improving.'

Homoeopathic philosophy has determined that real health is present when the mental, emotional and physical elements of a person are at one. As was mentioned earlier, it was this suppression of symptoms that created inherited miasms. Practice has shown that where physical symptoms are suppressed, the disease is driven inward and, more than likely, will manifest as mental or emotional symptoms. For example, it is interesting to note that usually schizophrenics do not suffer from many physical symptoms, but if their mental symptoms are suppressed, these will begin to manifest, probably, as a serious physical disease.

A homoeopath will look for what is known as the direction of cure. A return of old symptoms, a curative effect from above to below and from the innermost, dangerously affected organs to the outer skin layer and the extremities. A classically acknowledged example of this is that of the suppressed excema in a child, which later develops into asthma and subsequently, if again suppressed, into heart disease. When correctly treated, these symptoms will return in reverse order until the excema disappears forever.

Vaccination was mentioned earlier in the context of the United States where there is compulsory vaccination for children entering school. In the UK there is a growing trend to vaccinate against even the most common childhood illnesses such as measles. Granted there is risk to children of permanent damage from many illnesses but there is also the fact that the disease assists the process of building up the child's immune system and suppressing that process will not help their development and may even result in another kind of damage from the side effects of the vaccination.

There are many statistics that suggest that the acknowledged side effects of some vaccines at least equal the dangers of the disease, if not surpass them. However, there are few statistics that show what kind of suppressive damage, likely to increase the susceptibility to conduct disorder, might be occurring in the brain of the vaccinated child.

In his book Vaccination, Social Violence and Criminality Harris L Coulter, while acknowledging the reduction and eradication of many life-threatening diseases in adults, explores and condemns the practice of mass vaccination for the common diseases of childhood. In more severe cases of measles, mumps and whooping cough, these carry the danger of brain damage from encephalitis but he questions the practice of administering a vaccine which causes encephalitis in the immature immune system and identifies this widespread programme as a major cause of developmental disabilities in industrialised countries. The dangers are well enough acknowledged in the United States for pharmaceutical companies to lay aside a significant percentage of the cost of vaccines to create a fund to compensate brain damaged children.

Certainly it is common in homoeopathic practice to treat a healthy robust child who, after routine vaccination, becomes sleepless, listless, starts to head bang, experiences learning difficulties or becomes withdrawn. These are only some of the many symptoms that may manifest, of which a number could be said to fall under a diagnosis of early Conduct Disorder. It is possible to antidote the effects of these vaccines homoeopathically but, left untreated, they might well proceed to become an acquired miasm.

Clearly, both medical and homoeopathic evidence accepts that environmental factors play a large part, while homoeopathy acknowledges the role of disease, as well as vaccination as being contributory to behavioural changes.

Another contributory environmental factor that should not be ignored is food allergy. In some cases an individual may be so allergic to a type of food, as to become violent or completely unreasonable after its consumption. In his book Mental Illness and schizophrenia - The Nutrition Connection, Dr Carl Pfeiffer makes the case for the nutritional approach to many disorders. The term 'orthomolecular' was first coined by Nobel Prize winner, Linas Pauling who acknowledged the efficaciousness of treating mental disorders with nutrition. However, Dr Pfeiffer advocates the use of vitamin supplements in large doses, a course that would not be appropriate when undertaking homoeopathic treatment.

Food additives, or 'the E numbers', are now recognised as being a contributory factor in some cases of mental disorder. Ellen Rothera in her book Allergy and Environmental Illness, also mentions household cleaners, toiletries and other chemical concoctions as being possible allergens which might lead to the exhibition of any or several of the following symptoms that would fall into the Conduct Disorder category. These include short concentration span, restlessness, aggression, excitability, difficulty in relating to peers, rapid mood changes and outbursts of temper.

However, it is important to note that these environmental factors would have to produce a 'repeated and persistent pattern of behaviour' to qualify as symptoms of Conduct Disorder.

3

THE MIASMATIC INFLUENCE AT WORK

A study of the charts on 29 and 30 will show that a small selection of rubrics are common to many of the listed criteria in Conduct and Antisocial Personality Disorders. Those that have been selected feature in ten or more of the symptoms given in the two DSMIV criteria. Were all the symptoms to appear in any one individual, Conduct Disorder has the potential of fifteen and Antisocial Personality Disorder, seven. The potential number of symptoms in both disorders would total twenty-two. A total of ten, therefore, would indicate a core of behaviour which is relatively common to a typical sufferer from either disorder.

The importance of a remedy in any one rubric in Kent's repertory is indicated by black, italic or light type which numerically equal 3, 2 and 1 respectively. The remedies that arise are laid out in order of their importance from the rubrics which scored ten or over in the charts on pages 23 to 26. They are, in order of importance:

Anacardium, Lycopodium, Nux Vomica, Hyoscyamus, Lachesis, Mercurius, Phosphorus, Stramonium, Opium, Platina, Arsenicum Album, Natrum Muriaticum, Pulsatilla, Belladonna, Calcarea Carbonica, Conium, Cuprum Metallicum, Nitricum Acidum and Sulphur. The list continues with remedies that are also well indicated, though not quite as strong as the first group. These include: Aconite, Arnica, Aurum Metallicum, China, Cicuta Virosa, Helleborus, Natrum carbonicum, Phosphoric Acid, Agaricus, Ambra Grisea, Baryta Carb, Causticum, Guaicum, Hepar Sulphuris Calcarium, Ignatia and Veratrum Album. In the chart that follows, the

---

miasmatic influences as identified by Kent, Choudhury and Banerjea are noted.

REMEDY and Miasm	Source Dr S. K. BANERJEA	Source Dr H. CHOUDHURY	Source J. T. KENT
PLATINA			
Psora	1	2	2
Sycosis	1	0	0
Syphilis	0	1	0
ARSENICUM ALBUM			
Psora	3	3	3
Sycosis	3	0	0
Syphilis	1	2	3
NATRUM MURIATICUM			
Psora	3	3	3
Sycosis	3	0	0
Syphilis	1	0	0
PULSATILLA			
Psora	2	0	3
Sycosis	2	1	1
Syphilis	0	0	0
BELLADONNA			
Psora	1	2	1
Sycosis	0	0	0
Syphilis	0	0	0
CALCAREA CARBONICUM			
Psora	3	0	2
Sycosis	2	2	2
Syphilis	0	0	0
CONIUM			
Psora	2	2	2
Sycosis	2	1	1
Syphilis	1	2	2
CUPRUM METALLICUM			
Psora	1	2	2
Sycosis	0	0	0
Syphilis	0	0	0
NITRICUM ACIDUM			
Psora	2	3	2
Sycosis	3	3	3
Syphilis	3	3	3

REMEDY and Miasm	Source	Source	Source
	Dr S. K. BANERJEA	Dr H. CHOUDHURY	J. T. KENT
SULPHUR			
Psora	3	3	3
Sycosis	2	2	2
Syphilis	2	2	2
ACONITE			
Psora	0	0	1
Sycosis	0	0	0
Syphilis	0	0	0
ARNICA			
Psora	2	0	1
Sycosis	0	0	0
Syphilis	0	0	0
AURUM METALLICUM			
Psora	2	2	1
Sycosis	1	2	1
Syphilis	3	3	3
CHINA OFFICINALIS			
Psora	0	0	1
Sycosis	0	0	0
Syphilis	0	0	0
CICUTA VIROSA			
Psora	0	0	2
Sycosis	0	0	0
Syphilis	0	0	0
HELLEBORUS NIGER			
Psora	0	0	1
Sycosis	0	0	0
Syphilis	0	0	0
NATRUM CARBONICUM			
Psora	3	2	2
Sycosis	2	0	0
Syphilis	0	0	0
PHOSPHORIC ACID			
Psora	1	2	1
Sycosis	0	0	0
Syphilis	1	2	2

REMEDY and Miasm	Source	Source	Source
	Dr S. K. BANERJEA	Dr H. CHOUDHURY	J. T. KENT
AGARICUS MUSCARIUS			
Psora	0	2	3
Sycosis	1	2	2
Syphilis	0	0	0
AMBRA GRISEA			
Psora	1	2	2
Sycosis	0	0	0
Syphilis	0	0	0
BARYTA CARBONICUM			
Psora	2	2	2
Sycosis	2	2	2
Syphilis	1	0	0
CAUSTICUM			
Psora	3	0	3
Sycosis	2	2	2
Syphilis	2	0	0
GUAIACUM			
Psora	0	0	1
Sycosis	0	0	0
Syphilis	0	1	1
HEPAR SULPHURIS CALCARIUM			
Psora	3	3	1
Sycosis	2	2	1
Syphilis	3	2	2
IGNATIA AMARA			
Psora	0	0	1
Sycosis	0	0	0
Syphilis	0	0	0
VERATRUM ALBUM			
Psora	1	0	1
Sycosis	1	0	0
Syphilis	0	0	0

Once again, it is important to emphasise at this stage, that these remedies suggest a core to the disorders, but that each case is treated individually and the individual set of symptoms will dictate the eventual choice of remedy which may be <u>none</u> of those listed.

It is striking to note that Vermeulen in his Synoptic Materia Medica identifies almost all the remedies listed above as having strong affinities with the brain, the mind and the nerves. The exceptions are Mercury, Nitric Acidum, Calcarea Carbonica, Sulphur and Guaicum. However, on studying the mental symptoms of these remedies one can find aberrations that fit the mental picture of these disorders in each. Some of these are illustrated below:

MERCURIUS
Instability on all levels

CALCAREA CARBONICA
Mischievous, obstinate, full of fears, poor learner

NITRIC ACIDUM
Irritable, hateful, vindictive, quarrelsome.
No disposition to work

SULPHUR
Lazy, dull, obstinate, slothful

GUAICUM
Critical, despises everything, indolent, obstinate and fretful.

Returning to the miasmatic influences, to obtain a 'feel' for each of the miasms discussed, it is useful to return to its original disease source.

As mentioned earlier, Hahnemann identified the scabious eruption (204, The Organon) as the original disease source and named this miasm PSORA. When studying the symptoms of scabies it is seen to be an exquisitely itchy, very contagious skin complaint caused by the mite Sarcoptes scabei. It is characterised by a nighttime aggravation of the itching and the skin shows eruptive evidence of the mite which burrows under the skin. It is the liquid from the vesicles that causes infection of the surrounding area and on skin contact with other individuals.

The manifestation of this Psoric miasm is an internal itch with or without its attendant eruption on the skin. This disease can affect all spheres of the human economy, but for the purposes of this discussion, the mental state will be explored.

Known as the sensitising miasm, the mental symptoms of Psora include hypersensitivity to the slightest stimuli, extreme restlessness, irritability, mood swings, indolence, dissatisfaction, censorious. In the perverted state, Dr Banerjea describes Psora as the reprobate with a mind to commit evil. Inconsistency, deceit, and a craving to achieve unnecessary objects, selfishness without conscience, dishonesty, secrecy and wickedness all feature as symptoms of this miasm. Although they do have outbursts of anger, these are not accompanied by a desire to harm anyone or anything.

GONORRHOEA, which is the suppressed sexually transmitted disease that emerges as the SYCOTIC Miasm, presents in the male with a urethral discharge and painful urination. Five percent of carriers may be asymptomatic as opposed to the female who number 7%. In the female the features are not as pronounced, with there being the appearance of a slight vaginal discharge and pain on passing water. In general, the disease is characterised by its discharges, suggesting a state of excess.

When observing the miasm that arises from this disease state, the mental picture that emerges is also one of excess. In this miasm can be recognised many symptoms of the mind that correlate with the criteria for Conduct and Antisocial Personality Disorder.

A sycotic mind is cross and irritable given to fits of anger, but in this case there is a great predisposition to cruelty to people as well as animals which is unlike the psoric anger. However, two miasms combined, Sycosis and Psora, are seen to form the basis for criminal insanity. The person can be degenerate with a jealous and suspicious nature and is likely to find any means of excusing his actions. The sycotic personality is quarrelsome, crafty and deceitful, bent on mischief. Their many negative characteristics include mendacity, selfishness and they are amoral and devoid of feelings of affection towards others. A sycotic person seems to have the ability to manipulate another's mind and have the tendency to be very vindictive.

Combined with the syphilitic miasm, sycotic personalities are sullen and smouldering which reflects the essence of the syphilitic disease which is one of concealment. The first evidence of primary SYPHILIS is the appearance of a painless ulcer about a month after the disease has been contracted through sexual contact. It then heals and disappears while the patient may develop a non-itchy rash with a generalised lymphadenopathy and possible lesions around the anus.

The third stage, which can appear many years after the initial infection, manifests as gummata patches on the skin, mucous membranes, then finally, the degeneration develops in the spinal chord with a final deterioration of the mind into insanity. The whole picture of the disease is one of destruction and self-concealment while the process continues until it finally appears as more serious diseases many years later.

The picture of the syphilitic miasm is also one of hidden symptoms and destruction. They have a desire to kill. Their ideas are fixed and they are obstinate. The syphilitic personality keeps his problems to himself. He is restless, malicious, mischievous and hateful, destructive, perverted and dissolute. The syphilitic has no sense of duty or responsibility. The destruction of things, people and even himself can be executed without warning - more on an impulse, the person never having mentioned the thought to a soul. It is also interesting to note that the (physical) malignancies of this miasm are prone to present at the age of around 40. Like the disease itself, they develop undetected until a later stage. The final degeneration of the brain to complete madness is one of the end consequences of untreated syphilis.

In summary these miasms can be classified in this way. The immorality of the sycotic miasm represents its lack of internal control, its excesses. Although destructive, this is not its purpose. The syphilitic character is not as explosive as the sycotic but more calculating (as it is in its nature to become buried) and it is these types who can be found behind political crime and acts of genocide.

The psoric person is less of an active person, his keynotes are those of hypersensitivity and theorising without following through with action. So one can recognise the person that would plan but not carry out a crime.

Over the generations these miasms have been inherited or acquired and as a consequence they have become amalgamated and mutated to create other miasms such as that of Tuberculosis - the 'child' of syphilis and psora.

The charts featured on pages 38 to 40 illustrate the miasmatic influences affecting the remedies listed. No one inherited factor can be pinpointed as running through the core picture of the Conduct or Antisocial Personality Disordered individual. Rather, each of the three basic miasms already discussed appear in different remedies. In some of the remedies that arise, no miasms comes through. Taking as examples of these remedies, Aconite and Arnica, there might be an originating cause that may trigger the behaviour, in the case of Aconite, fright, and Arnica could be caused by a shock of some kind.

Although there are many remedies that are indicated in the illustrations given, they do not take account of the wide range of others that may well be appropriate to the individual casetaking. Those others that are likely to present themselves include Tarantula, Staphysagria and Thuja. However, this would suggest that there would be more emphasis on symptoms outside the core group which would make each of these remedies appropriate to that patient. There are also the nosodes (or remedies made from the original diseased matter by the homoeopathic process of dilution and succussion) of Syphilinum, Psorinum, Medhorrinum, Carcinosin and Tuberculinum. These might by administered as a remedy if the clinical picture called for one, otherwise, in the treatment of miasmatic cases, it will be necessary to give the appropriate nosode as an intercurrent remedy. If given as an intercurrent, this is in a different potency to the remedy chosen for the patient's symptom picture. This procedure will help open the way for the remedy to continue working towards cure.

In the final analysis it has to be stressed once again, that the basis of homoeopathy is the individual casetaking, and the above remedies are only a guide as to those that may be indicated.

4

THE CONCLUSIONS

Homoeopathy and orthodox medicine are in agreement that there is no one gene that causes criminal behaviour in children and adolescents. Both acknowledge that there is an argument for the predisposition to antisocial behaviour through either the genetic or miasmatic route and both arrive at conclusions which make a case for an environmental or arousing element that would set off a pattern of this kind of behaviour.

When looking at the arguments presented in the previous sections, it is possible to see a number of instances where homoeopathic philosophy reflects the findings for the case of inherited criminal tendencies, as set out by the scientific world. In the case of twin studies on schizophrenia, it was shown that there is a strong familial tendency towards this disorder. Medicine acknowledges the heritability of susceptibility to disease such as cancer and alcoholism, so there seems to be little reason to deny the possibility of inheriting behavioural characteristics. After all, what is schizophrenia other than a highly accentuated set of behavioural symptoms?

The findings of the Vietnam Era Twin Registry indicated that genetics were more likely to influence adult antisocial behaviour than juvenile behaviour - another scientific argument for the inheritance factor.

The evidence presented by Dr Mednick of a Danish study amongst adopted children, presents convincing statistics to argue the case for the viability of a genetic predisposition towards criminal behaviour. It also emphasises the necessity, in most cases, of there being exposure to an example - in this case the adoptive parents - to set off the cycle of behaviour in the child. This is something which is accepted by homoeopaths who acknowledge that if the miasm (let us call this a gene equivalent for the purposes of this argument) is latent, it may be aroused by an environmental factor. This may be due to a learned pattern of behaviour or some other reason, completely unrelated, that might trigger the biological tendency to this antisocial behaviour.

When referring to the 'completely unrelated trigger factor', disease, vaccination, food, chemicals, trauma and other factors can be included in this group.

It is interesting to note that homoeopathy acknowledges that a miasm, which can be created as a result of disease, trauma, and suppressive medication, can be grafted on the person. This then becomes a part of their constitution. It is then available for transmission to their progeny as the 50% gene contribution to the incipient embryo in the gene self-selection process vital to its (the gene's) survival, as well as the human's survival as a species.

The example of the rabid dog has been cited as a source of gene introduction through a route that does not involve reproduction. This virus enters the host and changes its behaviour and personality to serve the need of that virus to survive. However, the behaviour becomes characteristic of the person suffering from rabies, causing hydrophobia, biting, aggression, in a previously normal person. This disease will either result in the death of the carrier, or a cure leaving the patient with the 'grafted' effects of these migrating genes as part of their own constitution. (Worth noting is that Hydrophobinum/Lyssin is another remedy to consider in cases of antisocial behaviour).

In the light of the scientific and homoeopathic evidence put forward for the genetic inheritance of antisocial behaviour, homoeopathy would welcome these patients as suitable cases for treatment. Whether diagnosed with Conduct or Antisocial Personality Disorder brought about in this way, or aroused by environmental circumstances, the patient would benefit greatly from homoeopathic treatment which, I believe, is not incompatible with medical and scientific conclusions.

AFTERWORD

An idea which has grown more intriguing during the course of this research is the possible presence of adrenaline levels in those people who suffer from both the disorders as outlined in this project.

The hormones produced by the Adrenal Medulla - Epinephrine and Norepinephrine - are activated to prime the nervous system to cope with stress. Excess secretion of these hormones result in a prolonged state of fight or flight, increasing heart rate and respiration, decreasing metabolic and respiratory use of energy the surplus of which is then directed towards the muscles.

The possibility of using adrenaline as a remedy led to an enquiry into its homoeopathic symptom picture and it was found that the mental picture is not pronounced. Despondency and nervousness, lack of interest in anything, no ambition, aversion to mental work, cannot concentrate on thoughts and the absence of 'grit' were present in the mental provings of the Suprarenal Gland as a sarcode as described in Agrawal's Materia Medica of Glandular Medicines. This proving was made in 1904 and there may well be a case for re-proving the remedy in the light of changes that have taken place in the world in the last ninety years.

More recent research and documentaries are also demonstrating that an acquired tendency towards violence is becoming more prevalent in children exposed to TV, films and computer games with violent material, including the news. In one documentary a group of children unused to watching violent films or playing aggressive virtual games were grouped in a room and asked to watch the news while their responses were monitored. These children reacted much more strongly with an increased level of adrenaline than those watching in the other group who were used to viewing similar material. This suggests that children exposed to violent material become desensitised to its content and may develop a more aggressive tendency as a result.